Self-assessment Picture Tests

Medicine

Volume 4

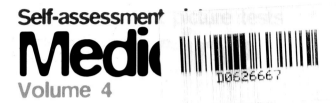

Pierre-Marc Bouloux

BSc MD FRCP

Reader in Endocrinology
Department of Endocrinology
Royal Free Hospital
London

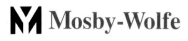

Mosby-Wolfe

London • Baltimore • Barcelona • Bogotá • Boston
Buenos Aires • Carlsbad, CA • Chicago • Madrid
Mexico City • Milan • Naples, FL • New York
Philadelphia • St. Louis • Seoul • Singapore
Sydney • Taipei • Tokyo • Toronto • Wiesbaden

Publisher:	**Richard Furn**
Development Editor:	**Jennifer Prast**
Project Manager:	**Linda Horrell, Jane Tozer**
Production:	**Gudrun Hughes**
Index:	**Angela Cottingham**
Layout:	**Lindy van den Berghe**
Cover Design:	**Greg Smith**

Published by Mosby–Wolfe, an imprint of Times Mirror International Publishers Limited

Printed in Italy by Imago

ISBN 0 7234 2467 5   Set ISBN 0 7234 2468 3

For full details of all Times Mirror International Publishers Limited titles, please write to Times Mirror International Publishers Limited, Lynton House, 7–12 Tavistock Square, London WC1H 9LB, England.

A CIP catalogue record for this book is available from the British Library.

Preface

Much of clinical practice consists of pattern recognition, and the ability to detect swiftly and interpret physical signs correctly is at the heart of the diagnostic process (and indeed a prequisite for passing clinical examinations!). In these four volumes, I have compiled 800 examples of common and not so common clinical problems covering wide areas of medicine. The format is simple, unambiguous and unpretentious: a photographic plate with a short question, or questions, relating to the physical sign or underlying diagnosis. The aim is to challenge the reader's diagnostic skills. I have annotated the answer in many cases to give the reader some background information about the condition illustrated. These volumes should be seen as an adjunct to existing illustrated textbooks of clinical medicine such as Forbes/Jackson *Color Atlas and Text of Clinical Medicine,* 2nd edition.

Acknowledgements

I would like to acknowledge the wonderful assistance given to me by the Department of Medical Illustrations at the Royal Free Hospital School of Medicine, and the excellent support of Miss Patsy Coskeran in assembling the material.

To Jane, Dominic, Matthew, Natalie and my late brother Alain

1 ▶
(a) What lesion is shown?
(b) List two biochemical
abnormalities associated
with this condition.

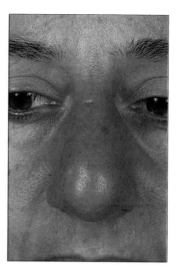

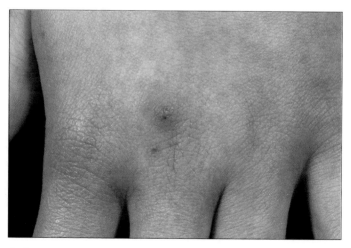

▲ 2
This is the hand of a lady who had unprotected sexual intercourse
some two weeks before. What is the most likely diagnosis?

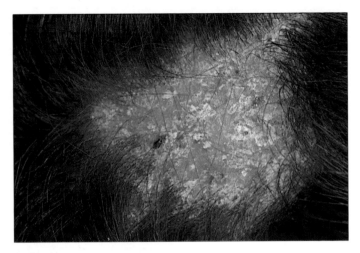

▲ 3
What is the most likely cause of this lesion?

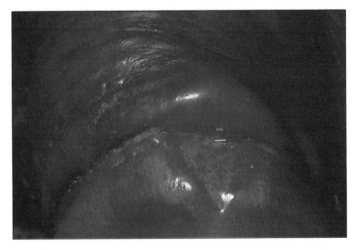

▲ 4
What is the most likely cause of this painless lesion, which occurred six weeks after sexual intercourse?

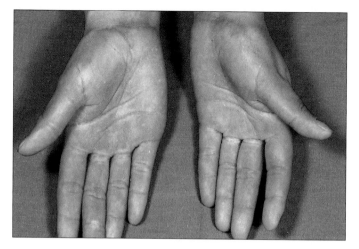

▲ 5
(a) What is the diagnosis?
(b) Cite one association.

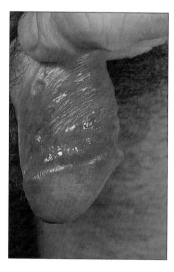

◀ ▼ 6
What diagnosis links the physical signs shown on the penis and in the eyes?

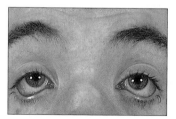

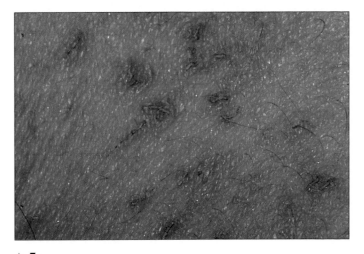

▲ 7
These lesions were pruritic. What is the diagnosis?

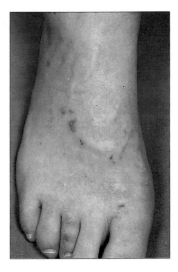

◄ 8
This lesion appeared to be migrating and was itchy. What is the most likely diagnosis?

9 ▶
This is the face of a child receiving immunosuppressive treatment. What is the likely causative organism?

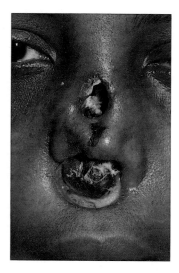

10 ▶
What is the most likely diagnosis?

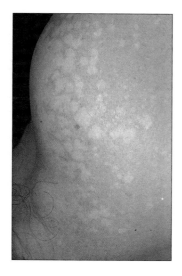

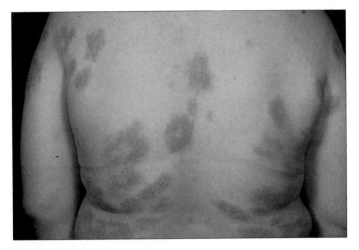

▲ 11
These lesions had been present for eight months. The patient also had nocturia and constipation. Suggest a unifying diagnosis.

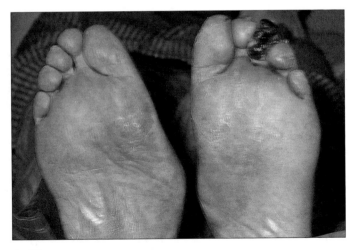

▲ 12
These are the feet of a diabetic patient. What physical sign is shown?

13 ▶

(a) What physical sign is shown?

(b) With what condition is it associated?

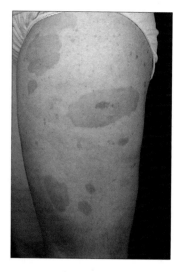

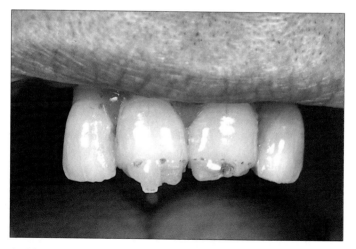

▲ **14**

(a) What physical sign is shown?

(b) With what condition is it associated?

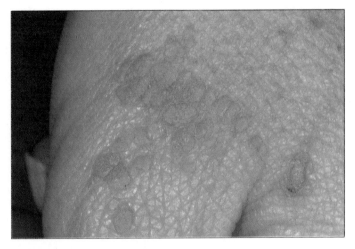

▲ 15
This patient was receiving azathioprine therapy. What is the most likely cause of these appearances?

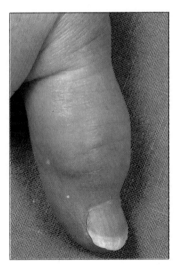

◀ 16
This patient has iritis. What is the most likely cause of this appearance?

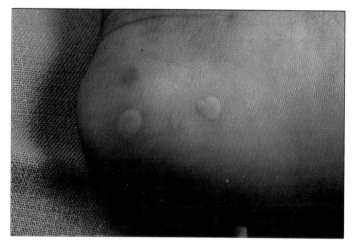

▲ 17
Lesions were also present in this patient's mouth. What is the most likely diagnosis?

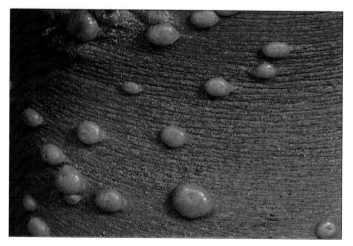

▲ 18
What is the diagnosis?

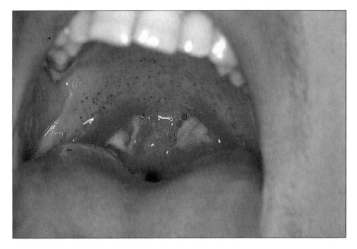

▲ 19
This patient was under investigation for a severe sore throat and abnormal liver function tests. What is the most likely diagnosis?

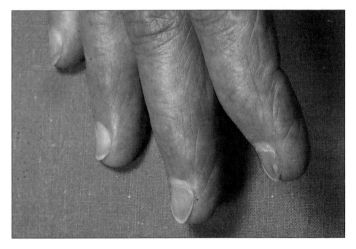

▲ 20
(a) What physical sign is shown?
(b) With what is it associated?

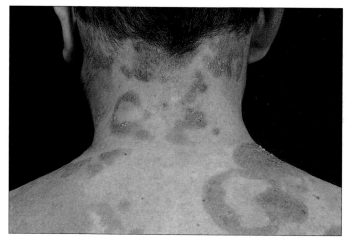

▲ 21
These lesions were present on a 45-year-old male. They began as itchy papules, and infiltrated plaques subsequently appeared. What is the most likely diagnosis?

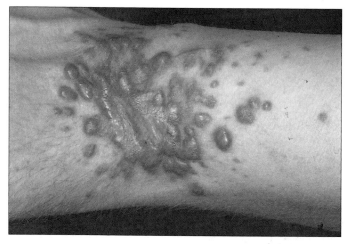

▲ 22
What is the diagnosis?

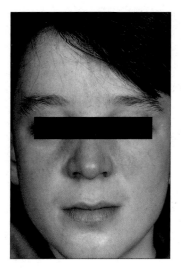

◀ 23
This patient presented with considerable proximal myopathy. What is the most likely diagnosis?

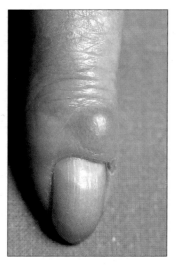

◀ 24
What is the diagnosis?

25 ▶

What is the most likely cause of
this chronic lesion?

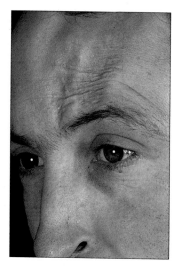

26 ▶

What physical sign is shown?

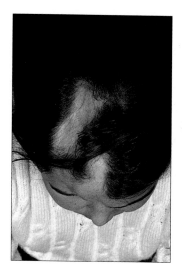

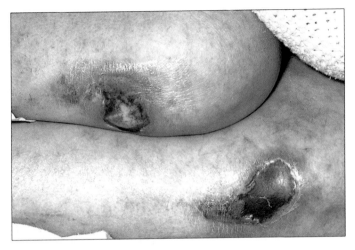

▲ 27
This patient was admitted comatose and diagnosed as having rhabdomyolysis. What lesions are shown?

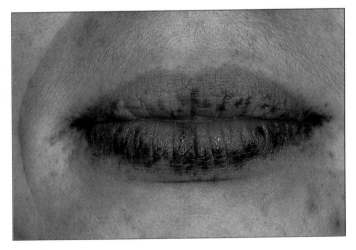

▲ 28
This patient was investigated for gastrointestinal bleeding. What is the likely diagnosis?

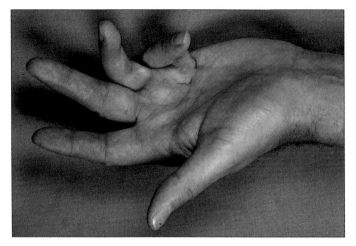

▲ 29
(a) What physical sign is shown?
(b) List two associations.

30 ▶
What myotome distribution
does this lesion have?

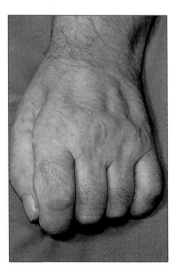

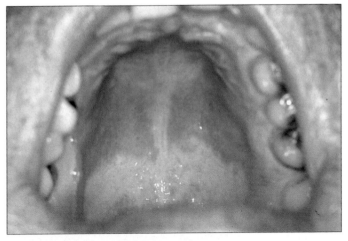

◄ ▲ 31
The physical signs
shown in these two
illustrations were
found in a patient
who was being
treated for a
chronic arthritic
condition. What is
the most likely
diagnosis?

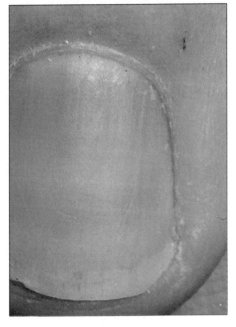

32 ▶
What is the diagnosis?

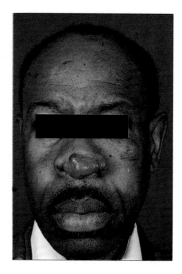

33 ▶
What is the diagnosis?

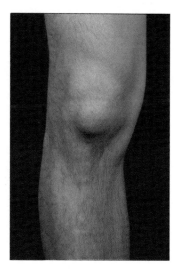

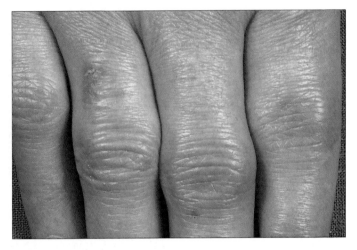

▲ 34

This patient had pericarditis and chronic renal failure. What is the most likely diagnosis?

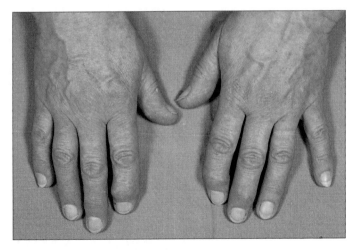

▲ 35

What is the most likely diagnosis?

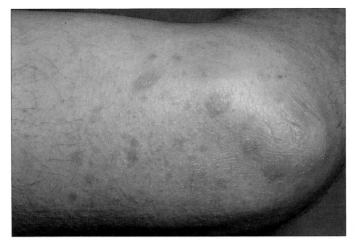

▲ 36
This rash was found in a young girl under treatment for arthritis and chronic uveitis. What is the most likely diagnosis?

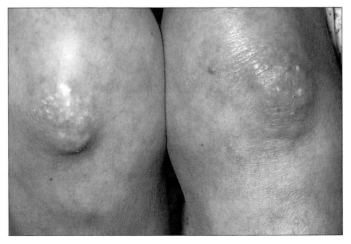

▲ 37
What is the most likely cause of this appearance?

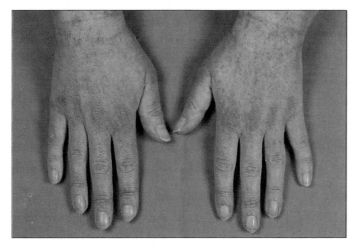

▲ 38

This patient was being investigated for weight loss and severe weakness. What is the most likely diagnosis?

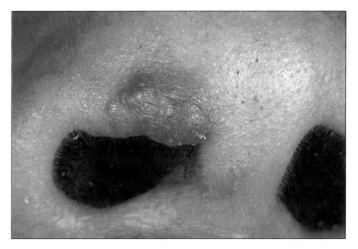

▲ 39

What is the most likely cause of this chronic lesion?

40 ▶

(a) What physical sign is shown?

(b) List two other physical signs that should be sought.

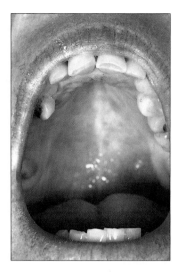

41 ▶

This patient was breathless. What is the likely unifying diagnosis?

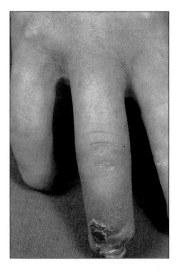

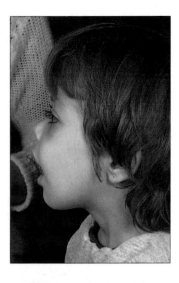

This patient was passing orange urine. Why?

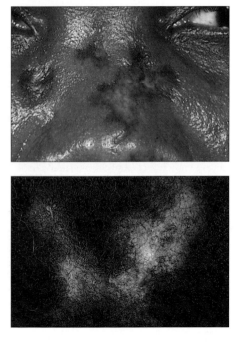

◀ ▼ 43
These two pictures depict a single condition. What is it?

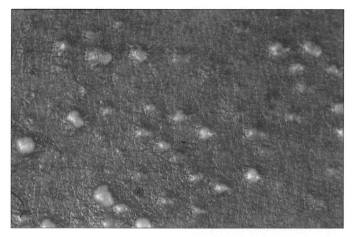

▲ 44

This man presented with a widespread pustular eruption associated with a high fever. There was considerable leucocytosis, but blood cultures were repeatedly negative. What is the most likely diagnosis?

45 ▶

What is the most likely cause of this appearance?

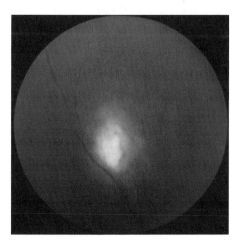

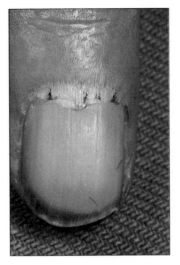

◀ **46**
What is the diagnosis?

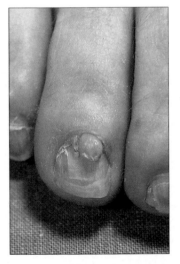

◀ **47**
What is the diagnosis?

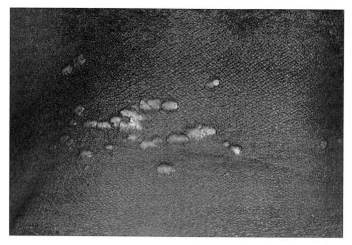

▲ 48

This patient had chronic uveitis. What is the most likely cause of this appearance?

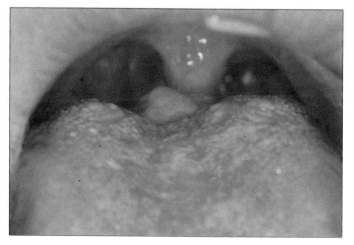

▲ 49

This lesion had been present since birth. What is the most likely diagnosis?

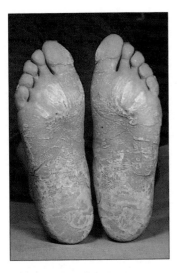

(a) What lesion is shown?
(b) Cite one association.

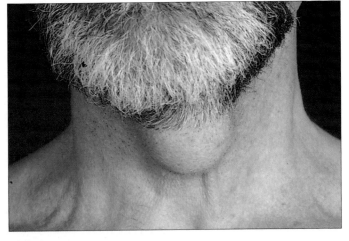

▲ 51
This lesion had been present since birth, but was getting progressively larger. What is the most likely diagnosis?

What is the diagnosis?

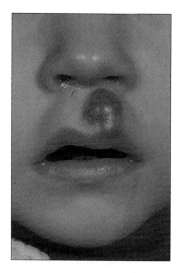

53 ▶
What diagnosis do
these two pictures
suggest?

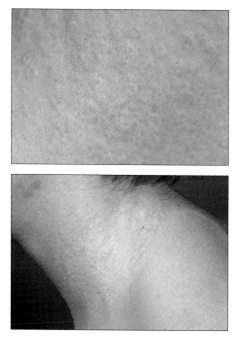

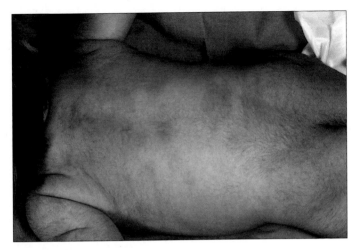

▲ 54
What lesion is shown?

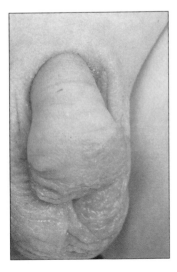

◄ 55
This mother was worried about the direction of her son's urinary stream. What is the diagnosis?

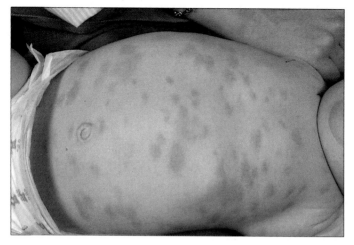

▲ 56

This child's mother noticed blistering eruptions and occasional lightly pigmented papules in the skin, which swelled when scratched or after a hot bath. What is the most likely diagnosis?

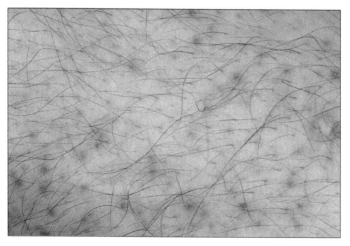

▲ 57

What is the diagnosis?

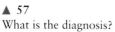

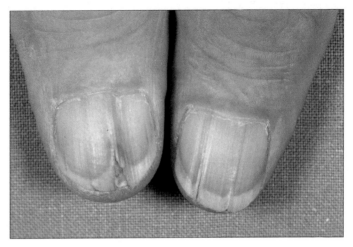

▲ 58
What is the diagnosis?

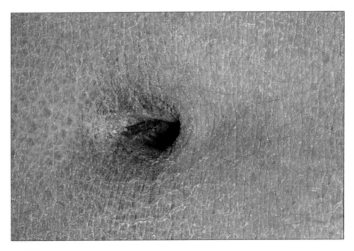

▲ 59
This lesion had been present for over 15 years. What is the most likely diagnosis?

60 ▶

The appearance of the legs had not changed substantially since childhood. What is the most likely diagnosis?

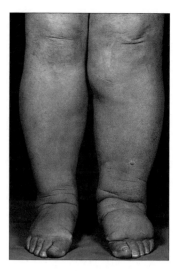

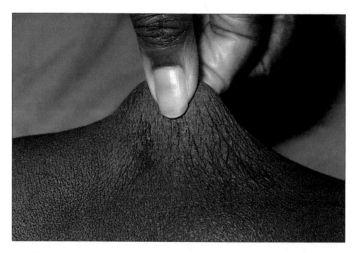

▲ **61**

(a) What physical sign is shown?

(b) What is the underlying diagnosis?

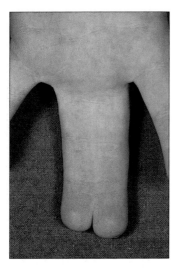

◀ 62
(a) What physical sign is shown?
(b) Cite one association.

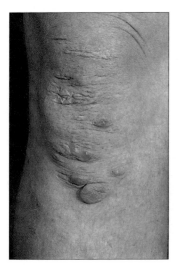

◀ 63
This patient was under investigation for a chronic anaemia. What is the most likely diagnosis?

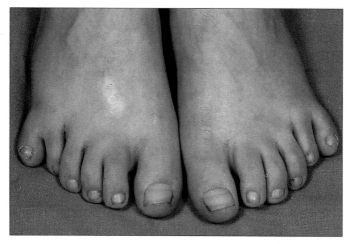

▲ 64
What physical sign is shown?

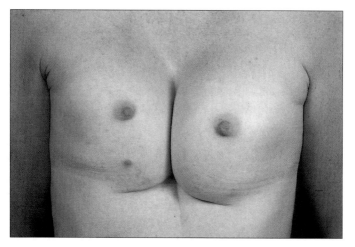

▲ 65
What physical sign is shown?

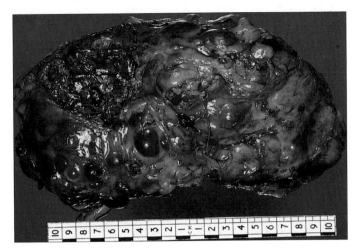

▲ 66
What is the diagnosis?

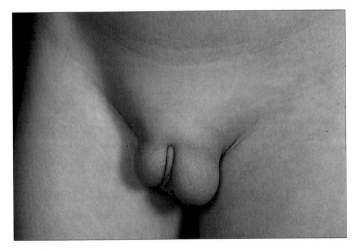

▲ 67
What may cause a swelling in these ambiguous genitalia?

68 ▶

These lesions were intensely itchy, particularly after hot baths. What is the most likely diagnosis?

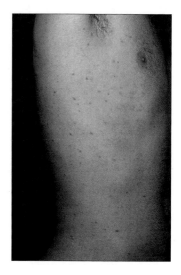

69 ▶

What is the diagnosis?

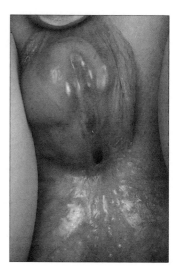

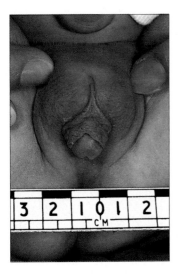

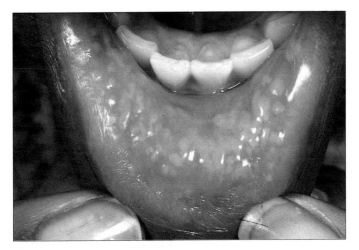

◀ 70
These are the genitalia of a patient who was XX. The child's parents were related. What diagnosis should be thought of?

▲ 71
What are these lesions?

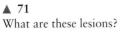

72 ▶
What physical sign is shown?

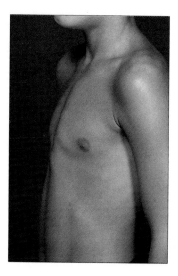

73 ▶
What is the most likely
underlying cause of these
appearances?

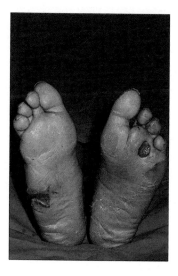

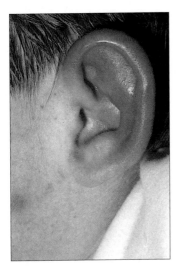

◀ 74

This man complained of a sore ear, first starting on one side, and then affecting the other side. What is the diagnosis?

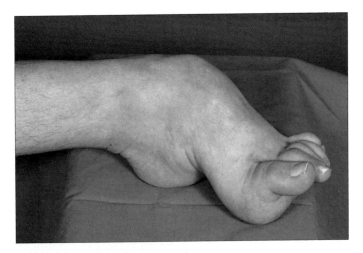

▲ 75

This is the foot of a man with a long-standing neurological disturbance that first affected his legs and was then associated with dysarthria. What is the most likely diagnosis?

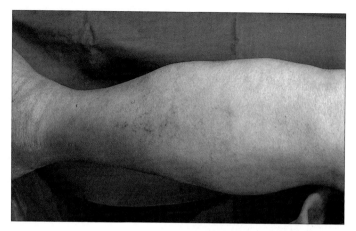

▲ 76
This is the leg of a patient being treated for heart failure.
(a) What is the most likely diagnosis?
(b) Cite one biochemical abnormality.

77 ▶
This man recently underwent a
bone marrow transplant. What
is the most likely diagnosis?

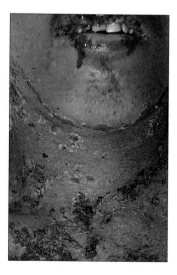

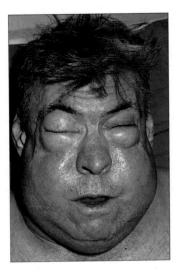

◀ 78
This is the appearance of a man following a road traffic accident. What is the most likely diagnosis?

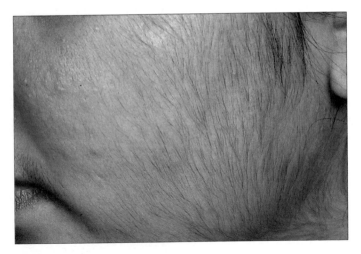

▲ 79
This patient had received a kidney during a transplant operation. What is the most likely cause of this appearance?

80 ▶

This man was receiving
treatment for a chronic
dysrhythmia. What is the most
likely cause of this appearance?

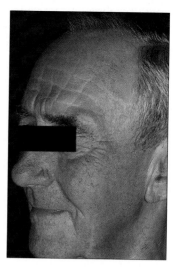

81 ▶

This is the fundal
appearance of an
asymptomatic
patient. What is the
diagnosis?

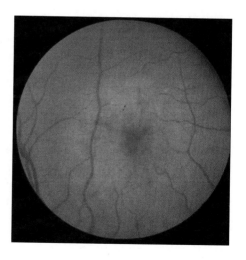

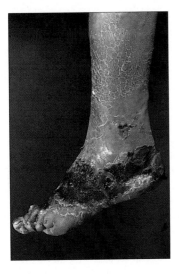

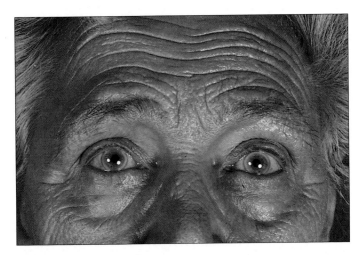

◄ 82
This is the foot of a man who
had been rescued from a
mountain expedition. What is
the diagnosis?

▲ 83
This is the appearance of a patient who had been taking eye drops
over a 20-year period. What is the most likely diagnosis?

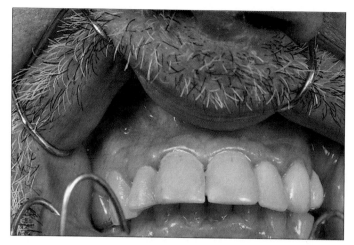

▲ 84

This man was under investigation for a sideroblastic anaemia. He was an artist. What is the likely diagnosis?

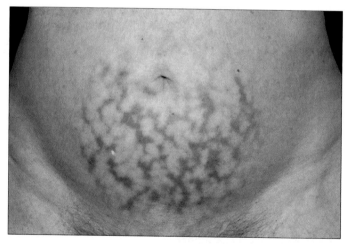

▲ 85

(a) What physical sign is shown?

(b) What symptom is likely to be associated with this physical sign?

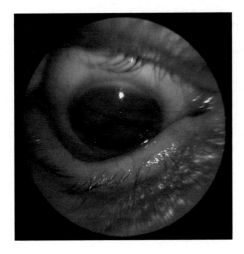

◄ 86
This is the eye of a patient who suffered from monocular diplopia. What physical sign is shown?

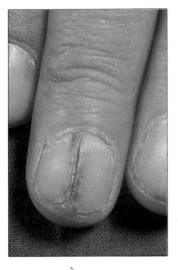

◄ 87
What is the diagnosis?

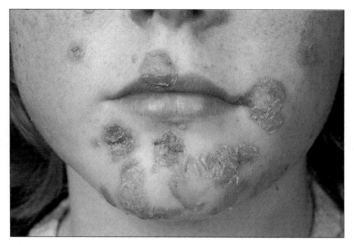

▲ 88
What is the diagnosis?

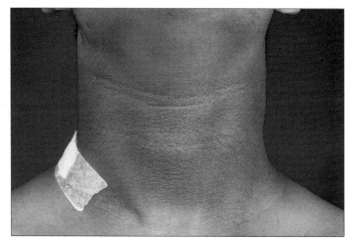

▲ 89
This patient was being treated for diabetes mellitus. What is the physical sign shown?

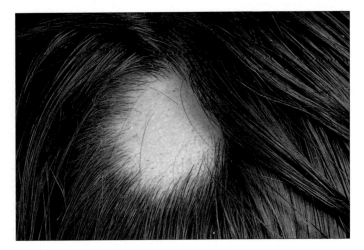

▲ 90

This patient developed a bald patch over the course of one week.
(a) What is the diagnosis of this acute lesion?
(b) What is the treatment?

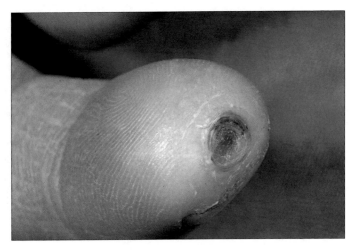

▲ 91

This patient had severe Raynaud's phenomenon and a history of dysphagia. What is the most likely diagnosis?

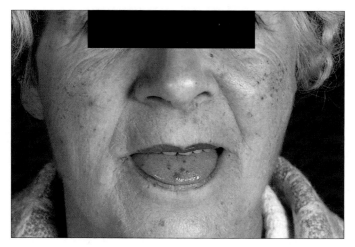

▲ 92

This lady had had several episodes of anaemia. What is the diagnosis?

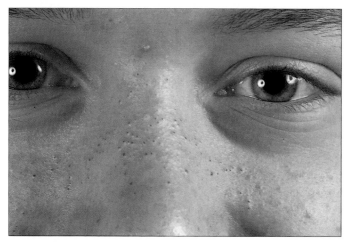

▲ 93

(a) What physical sign is shown?
(b) List two treatments to improve this appearance.

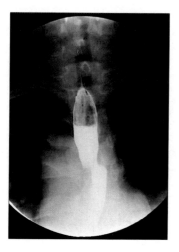

This patient had long-standing dysphagia, but was otherwise completely well. What is the most likely cause of this appearance?

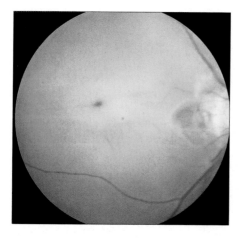

◀ 95
What is the diagnosis?

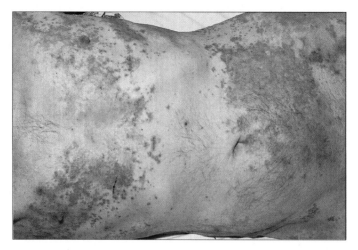

▲ 96

This eruption was present in a man with severe wasting and hyperglycaemia, and who was in a gross catabolic state. What is the most likely diagnosis?

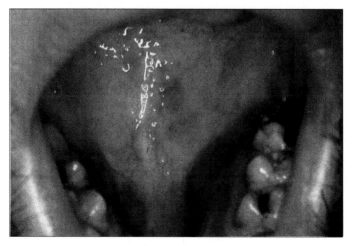

▲ 97

This homosexual man was being treated for severe weight loss. What is the diagnosis?

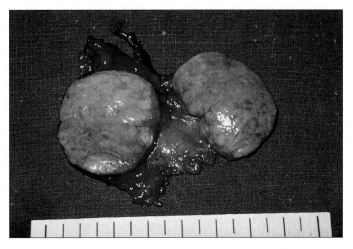

▲ 98

This is a resection specimen from a patient with hypertension and hypokalaemia. What is the diagnosis?

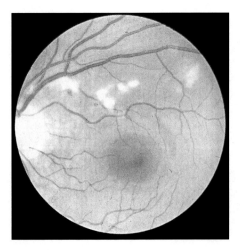

◄ 99

This is the fundal appearance of a patient on an intensive care unit following a major road traffic accident. What is the most likely cause of this appearance?

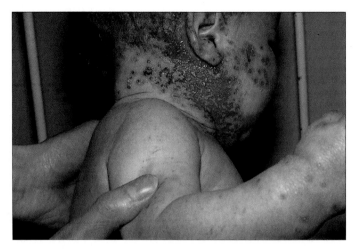

▲ 100
This child had severe eczema. What lesion is shown?

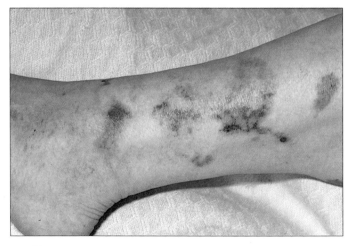

▲ 101
This patient had weight loss, a fever of unknown origin, and these lesions which all ulcerated. What is the most likely diagnosis?

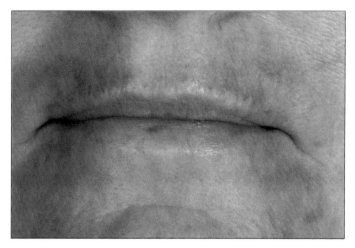

▲ 102
This patient had life-long iron-deficiency anaemia. What diagnosis should be considered?

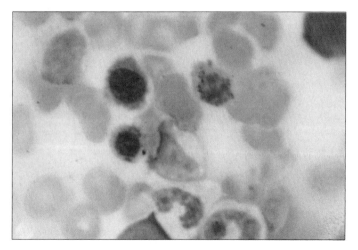

▲ 103
This is a bone marrow aspirate that has been stained for iron. What is the diagnosis?

104 ▶
What causes this
appearance?

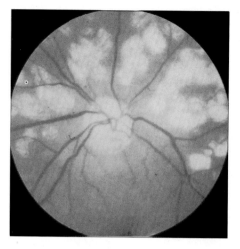

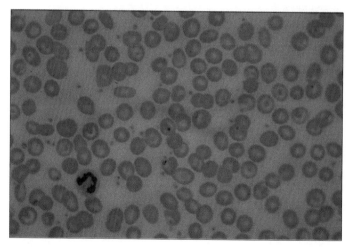

▲ **105**

(a) What morphological abnormalities of red cells are shown here?

(b) List three associations.

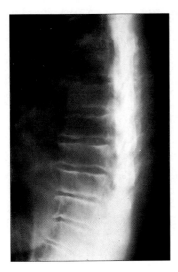

◀ 106
What is the most likely
diagnosis?

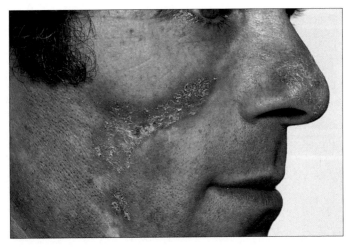

▲ 107
What is the most likely cause of this appearance?

108 ▶
What abnormality
is demonstrated on
this fluorescein
angiogram?

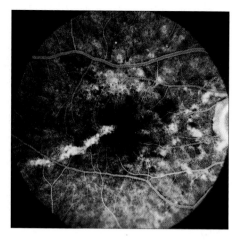

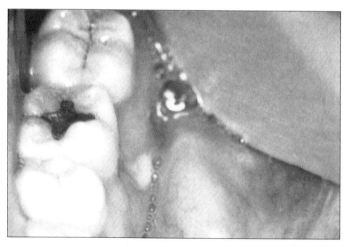

▲ 109
This lesion was found in the mouth of a patient with diabetes
insipidus, who also had pulmonary abnormalities. What is the
most likely diagnosis?

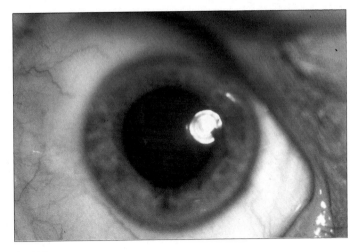

▲ 110
This patient was under investigation for severe malnourishment.
(a) What lesion is shown?
(b) What is the most likely diagnosis?

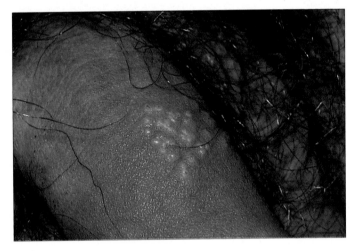

▲ 111
What is the diagnosis?

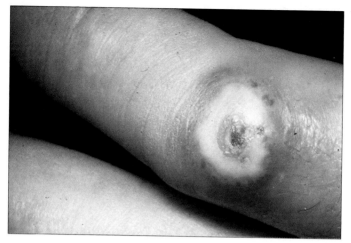

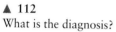
What is the diagnosis?

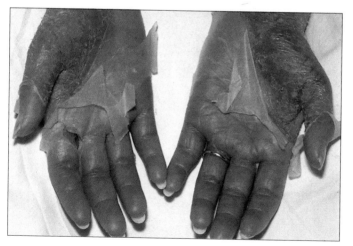

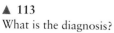
What is the diagnosis?

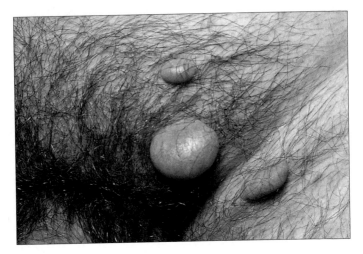

▲ 114

These lesions had been present since birth. What is the diagnosis?

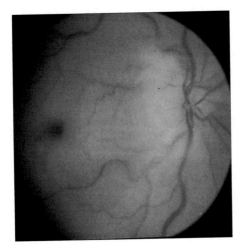

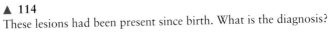

◄ 115

This patient complained of sudden loss of vision. What is the diagnosis?

116 ▶
What is the most
likely diagnosis?

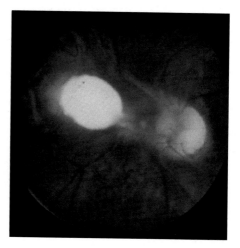

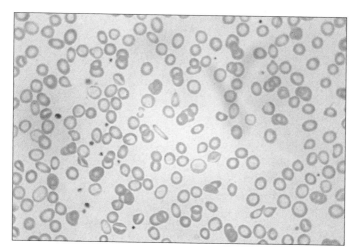

▲ 117
What is the likely diagnosis based on this blood film appearance?

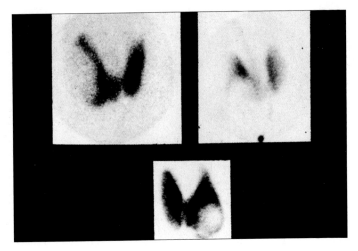

▲ 118
What lesions are shown on these three technetium scans of the thyroid?

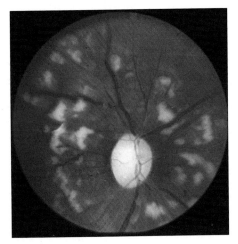

◄ 119
This is the fundal appearance of a 19-year-old negroid female.
(a) What physical sign is shown?
(b) What is a common association?

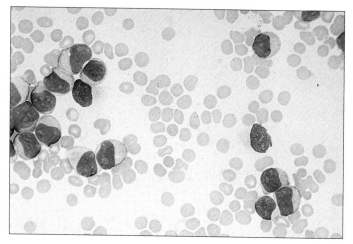

▲ 120
What is the diagnosis based on this blood film?

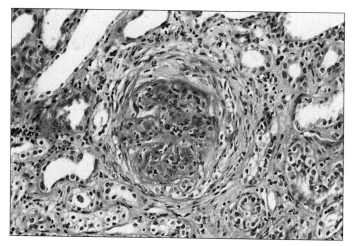

▲ 121
This is a renal biopsy from a patient with haematuria and heavy proteinuria. What is the diagnosis?

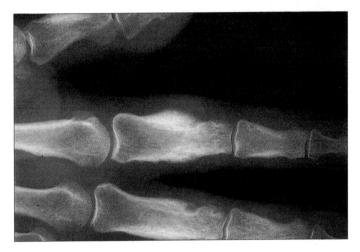

▲ 122
This patient had lost weight and was clubbed. What is the most
likely cause of this appearance?

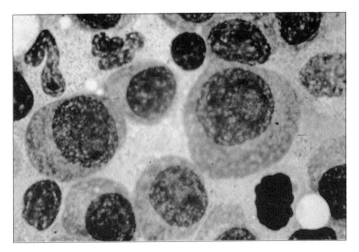

▲ 123
This is the bone marrow of a man with gross anaemia. What is the
diagnosis?

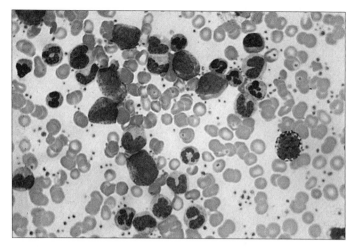

▲ 124
This is the blood film of a patient who had a three-year elevated
white cell count. What is the diagnosis?

125 ▶
What is the most
likely inference that
can be made from
this appearance?

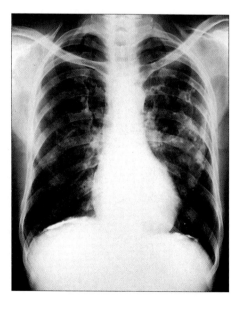

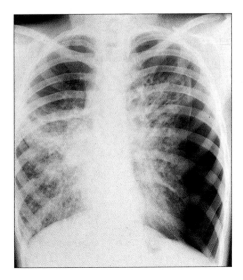

◀ **126**
This patient, with a chronic chest complaint, suddenly became very breathless. What is the most likely diagnosis?

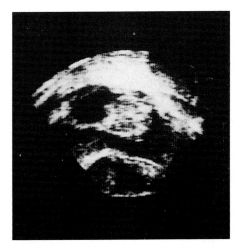

◀ **127**
This patient presented with a sudden loss of consciousness. What echocardiographic abnormality is demonstrated?

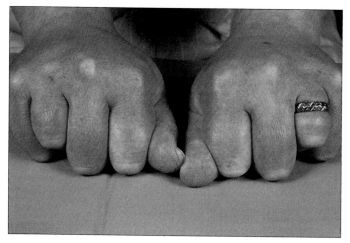

▲ 128
(a) What physical sign is shown?
(b) Cite one associated biochemical abnormality.

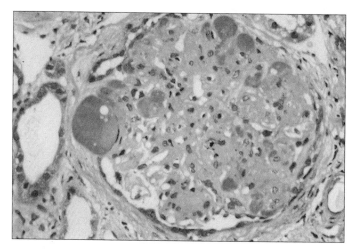

▲ 129
This is the renal biopsy from a patient with heavy proteinuria.
What is the diagnosis?

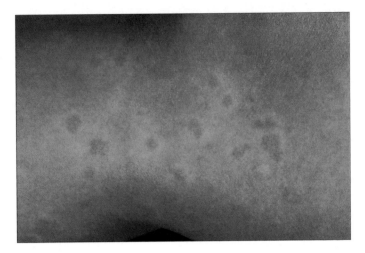

▲ 130
This is the skin of a thyrotoxic patient. What abnormality is shown?

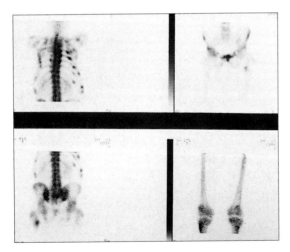

▲ 131
This is the bone scan of a patient complaining of aches and pains. What is the diagnosis?

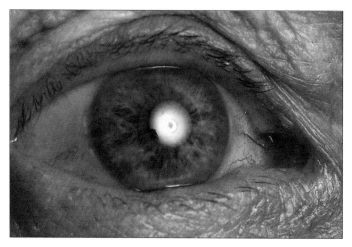

▲ 132
This patient was under investigation for nocturia. What physical sign is shown (ignore the central flash gun artefact)?

133 ▶
(a) What abnormality is shown?
(b) What physical sign should be sought?

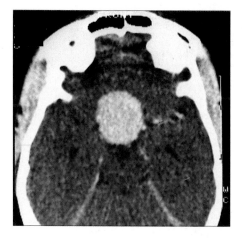

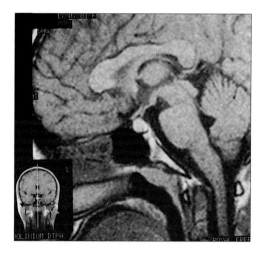

◄ **134**

(a) What investigation is shown?

(b) What abnormality is present?

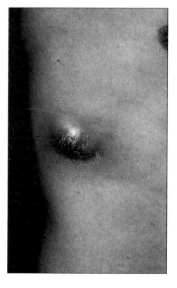

◄ **135**

This man was known to have a pleural effusion, had lost weight and had been pyrexial for over three months. What physical sign is shown?

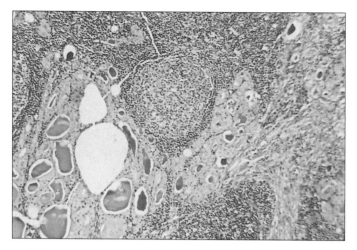

▲ 136
This is the histology of a lump removed from the neck. What is the
diagnosis?

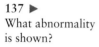
137 ▶
What abnormality
is shown?

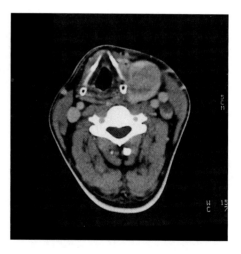

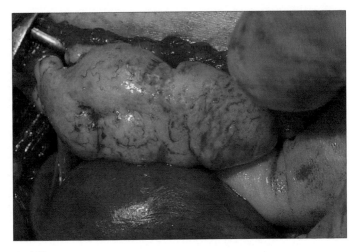

▲ 138

This is the ovarian appearance of a patient with hirsuties. What is the diagnosis?

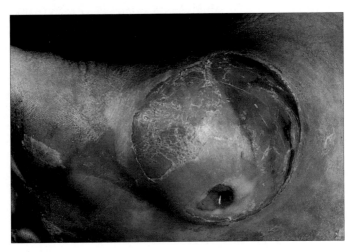

▲ 139

What is the diagnosis?

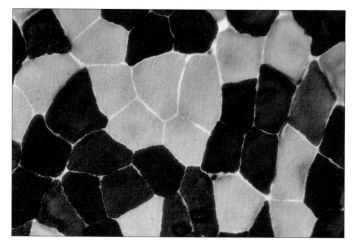

▲ 140
Comment on this biopsy appearance.

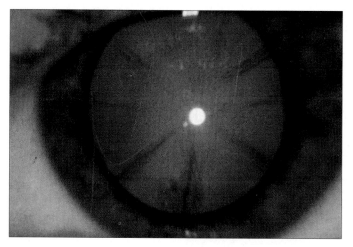

▲ 141
This man is diabetic. What ocular abnormality is shown?

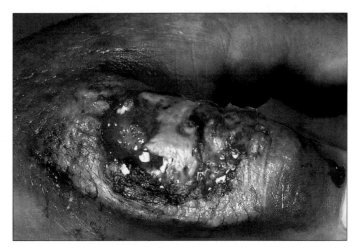

▲ 142
This patient had multiple lesions, like this, and also had weight loss from a chronic diarrhoeal illness. What is the diagnosis?

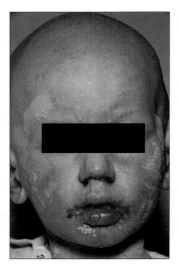

◀ 143
This child had a chronic enteropathic illness. What is the most likely cause of this appearance?

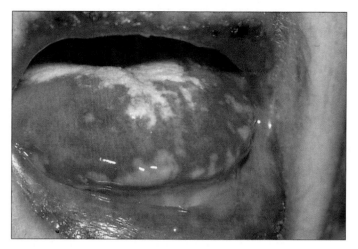

▲ 144
This appearance occurred one week after starting antibiotics.
What is the most likely diagnosis?

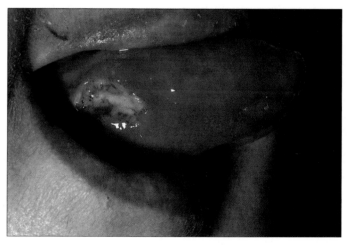

▲ 145
This patient also had genital ulcers and a sore eye. What is the
diagnosis?

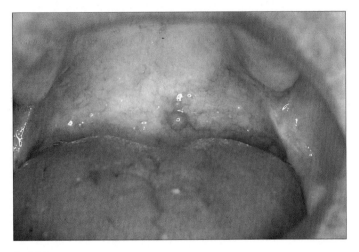

▲ 146
This patient had numerous bullous lesions over the buttocks and legs. What is the most likely diagnosis?

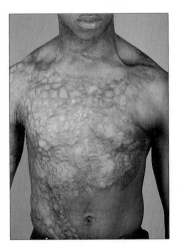

◄ 147
What is the most likely cause of this appearance?

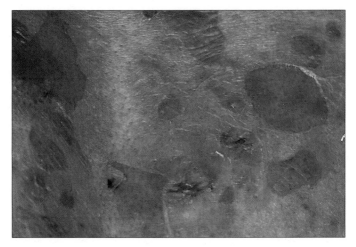

▲ 148

This patient had recently started treatment with a disease-modifying drug for rheumatoid arthritis. What is the most likely cause of this eruption?

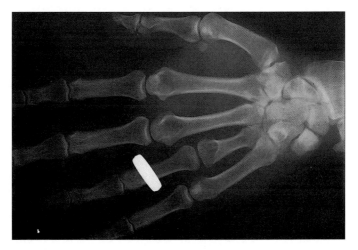

▲ 149

(a) What abnormality is shown?
(b) List two associations.

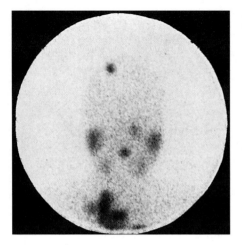

◀ 150
This man underwent this specialized investigation for a diagnosis of secondary hypertension. What is the most likely cause of this appearance?

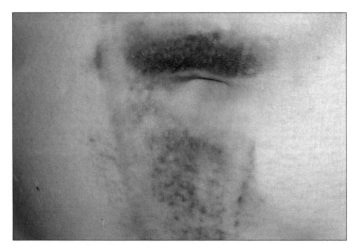

▲ 151
This patient fell on the ward and rapidly became anaemic. What is the most likely cause of this appearance?

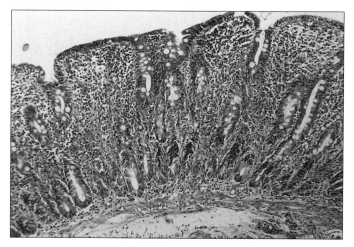

▲ 152

This is a small intestine biopsy from a patient with a distended abdomen and weight loss. What is the most likely cause?

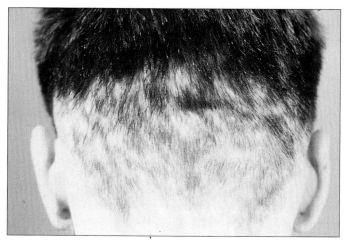

▲ 153

This sailor was under investigation for lymphadenopathy. What is the most likely cause?

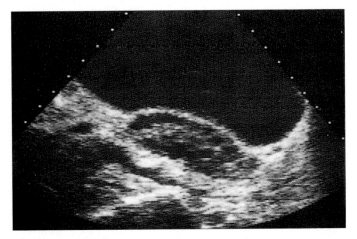

▲ 154

(a) What investigation is shown?
(b) What is the diagnosis?

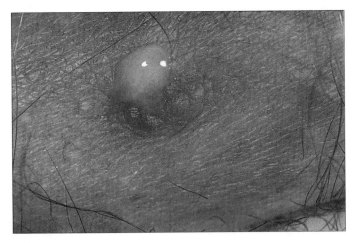

▲ 155

This is the nipple of a man. What are two possible causes for this physical sign?

156 ▶
What is the most likely cause of this appearance?

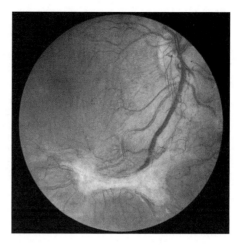

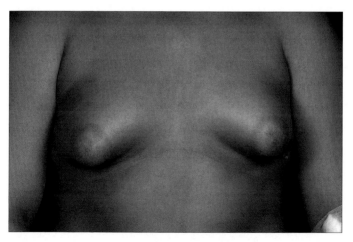

▲ **157**
This obese Afro-Caribbean boy was very conscious about his appearance.
(a) What physical sign is shown?
(b) What investigations are appropriate?

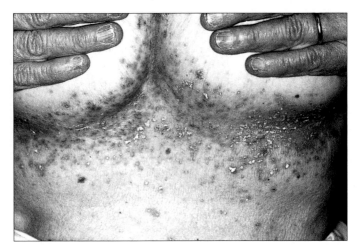

▲ 158
What is the cause of this appearance?

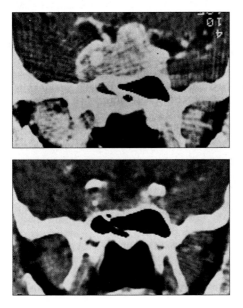

◄ ▼ 159
What treatment has probably been given to cause the change in appearance from the upper to the lower panel?

160 ▶

This man experienced occasional fits. What is the diagnosis?

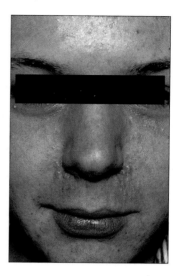

161 ▶

This patient had a scar in the neck. What is the most likely diagnosis?

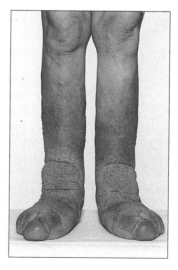

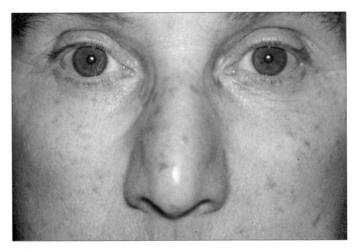

▲ 162
What is the diagnosis?

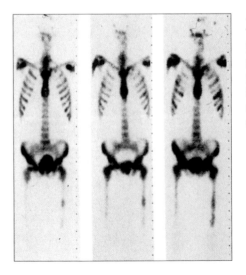

◀ 163
This patient was being investigated for a raised alkaline phosphatase. What is the most likely cause of this appearance?

164 ▶
What is the
diagnosis?

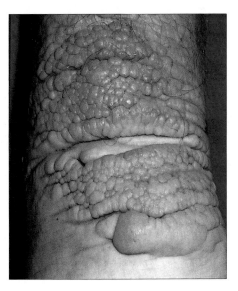

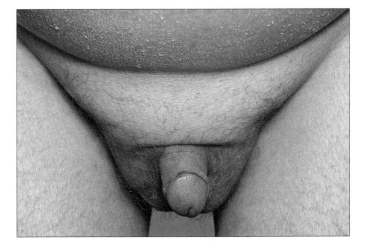

▲ 165
This man was 57 years' old and had failed to go through puberty.
What is the most likely diagnosis?

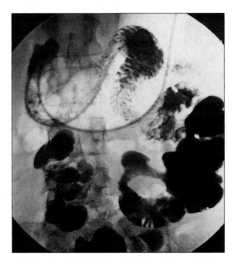

◀ **166**
This patient was being investigated for cramping abdominal pain, diarrhoea, and weight loss. What abnormality is present?

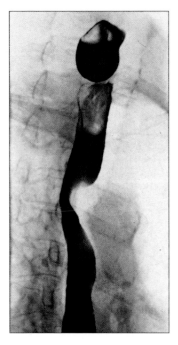

◀ **167**
This is a barium swallow. What is the most likely symptom with which the patient presented?

168 ▶

This patient had previously
been thyrotoxic. What is the
diagnosis?

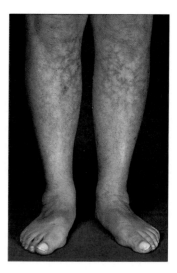

169 ▶

This patient was under
investigation for insomnia and
generalized weakness. What is
the most likely diagnosis?

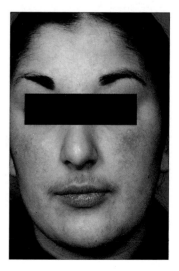

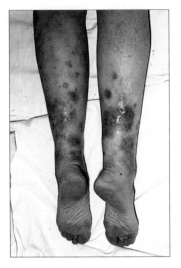

◀ 170
What is the most likely diagnosis?

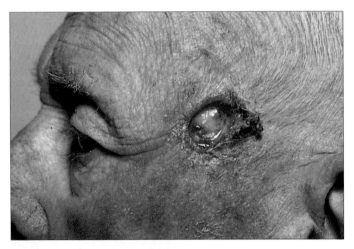

▲ 171
What is the diagnosis?

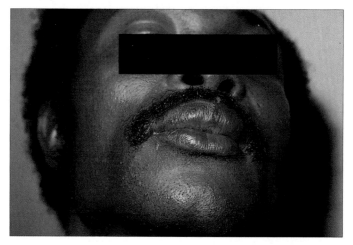

▲ 172
This man was using regular aperients. What lesion is shown?

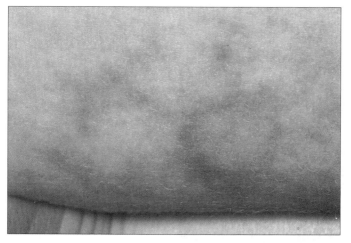

▲ 173
What lesion is demonstrated?

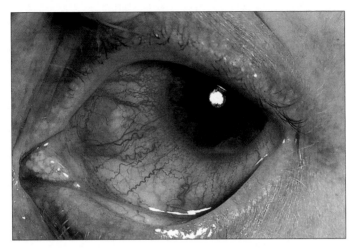

▲ 174
What is the most likely cause of this sore red eye?

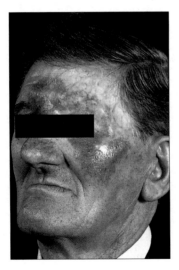

◄ 175
What is the most likely cause of this appearance?

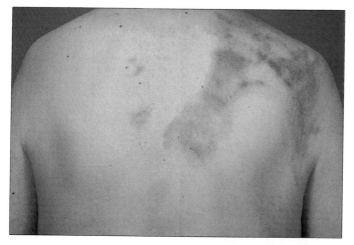

▲ 176

This man has diabetes mellitus. What is the most likely cause of these lesions?

177 ▶

This is the fundal appearance of a patient with fading visual acuity. What is the diagnosis?

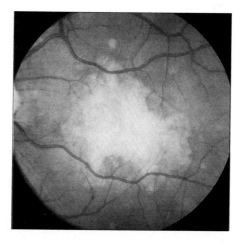

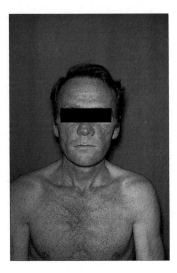

This patient also had a peripheral neuropathy. What is the most likely cause of this appearance?

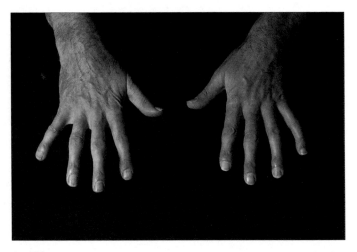

▲ 179
(a) What abnormality is shown in these hands?
(b) List two associations.

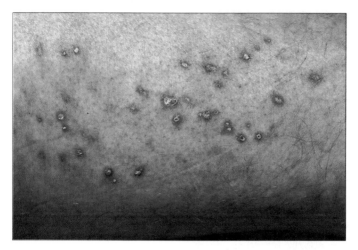

▲ 180
What is the likely cause of these multiple calcific lesions?

181 ▶
What is the most likely cause of
this appearance?

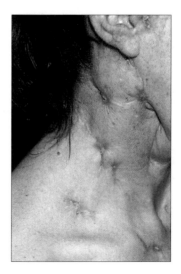

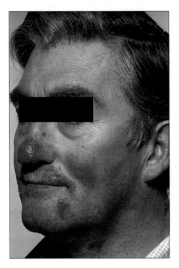

◀ 182
What is the most likely cause of this appearance?

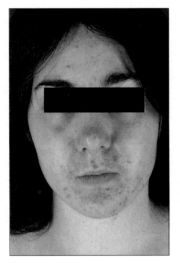

◀ 183
What is the most common cause of this abnormality?

184 ▶
List two
abnormalities.

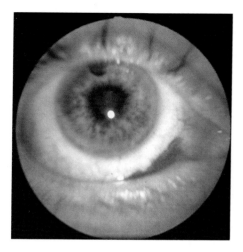

185 ▶
What is the likely cause of this
young man's short stature?

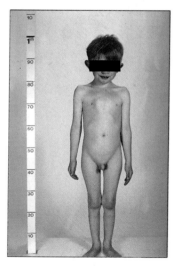

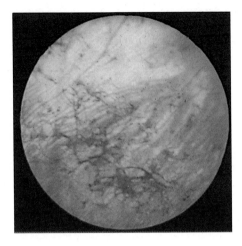

◀ 186
This is the appearance of the fundus of a patient who was in a long-term psychiatric ward. What is the most likely cause of this appearance?

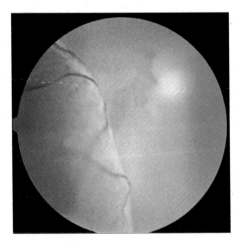

◀ 187
What is the diagnosis?

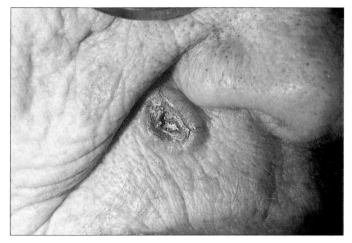

▲ 188
What is the diagnosis?

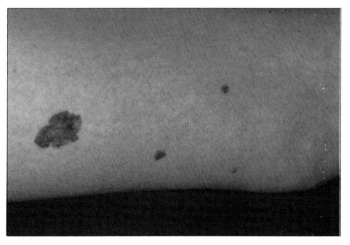

▲ 189
What is the most likely cause of this appearance?

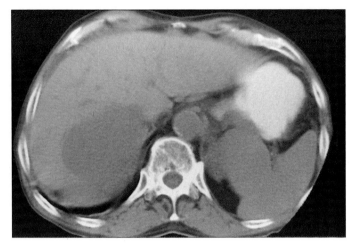

▲ 190
What is the most likely cause of this computerized tomography (CT) scan appearance?

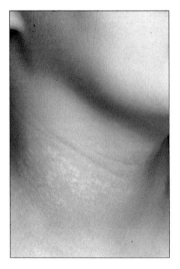

◄ 191
What is the most likely cause of this appearance?

192 ▶

What is the most
likely cause of this
appearance?

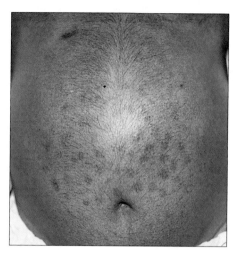

193 ▶

(a) What physical sign is
shown?
(b) Does this physical sign ever
occur under physiological
conditions?

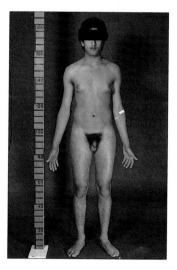

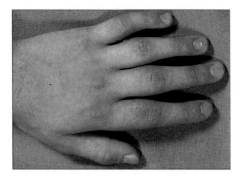

◀ 194
These are the hands of an 11-year-old patient with a rash, a fever, and a pain in the neck. What is the most likely diagnosis?

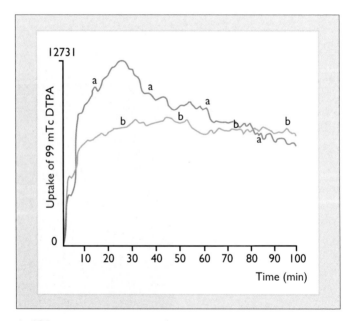

▲ 195
(a) What investigation has been performed on the kidneys?
(b) What abnormality is shown?

196 ►

This man had severe behavioural abnormalities. With what chromosomal abnormality is this associated?

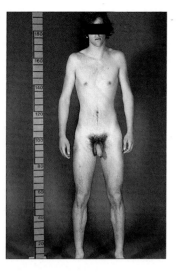

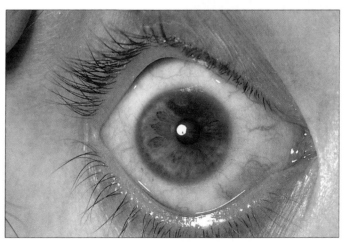

▲ **197**

What physical sign is shown?

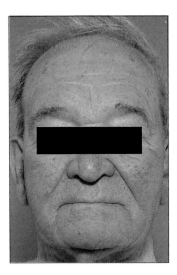

◀ 198
This man was admitted to casualty following a fall in the street. What diagnosis is suggested by his appearance?

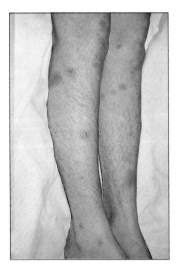

◀ 199
What is the most likely cause of this appearance?

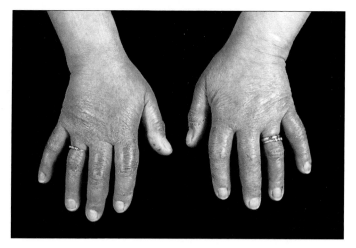

▲ 200
These are the hands of a traffic warden. What is the diagnosis?

1   (a) Lupus pernio in a patient with sarcoidosis.
    (b) Serum angiotensin-converting enzyme (ACE) levels should be measured,
    and the patient may have hypercalciuria.

2   Gonococcal infection. An early arthritis–dermatitis syndrome may occur
    in disseminated gonococcal infection, and is typically followed by a joint
    localization stage. In the early phase, migratory tenosynovitis and arthralgias
    may occur, as well as a papular or pustular skin lesions.

3   Ringworm infection of the scalp.

4   Primary chancre of syphilis.

5   (a) Hyperkeratosis palmaris (tylosis).
    (b) This may be associated with oesophageal carcinoma.

6   Reiter's syndrome. This consists of conjunctivitis, urethritis (or cervicitis
    in females), arthritis, and characteristic mucocutaneous lesions. *Chlamydia
    trachomatis* has been recovered from the urethra of up to 70% of men with
    untreated non-diarrhoeal Reiter's syndrome and associated urethritis.

7   Scabies.

8   Cutaneous larva migrans. In *Strongyloides stercoralis* infection, the
    migration of larvae under the skin is accompanied by urticarial weals
    overlying their course. This condition, called cutaneous larva migrans,
    affects most chronically infected patients from time to time. Larvae, where
    they penetrate the skin, cause pruritus.

9   *Aspergillus* infection.

10 Pityriasis versicolor.

11 Cutaneous sarcoidosis. The constipation and nocturia were associated with
    hypercalcaemia.

12 Bilateral Charcot's joints.

13 (a) Café-au-lait spots.
    (b) These are associated with neurofibromatosis.

14 (a) Hutchinson's teeth.
    (b) These are associated with congenital syphilis.

15 Cutaneous planar warts.

16 Sarcoidosis. The bony changes are probably associated with lupus pernio. The bony appearances are of two sorts: a lattice-like pattern of multiple rarefactions in a diffusely expanded phalanx, or localized, rounded, or oval rarefactions suggesting unilocular or multilocular cysts.

17 Hand, foot, and mouth disease. This is sometimes described as vesicular dermatitis with exanthema. The pharyngeal ulcers that are often seen in the mouth in this Coxsackie virus infection are less severe than in herpangina. There is a typical vesicular eruption on the hands and feet, and sometimes in small children, on the buttocks.

18 Molluscum contagiosum. The umbilicated lesions are clearly seen.

19 Glandular fever (infectious mononucleosis).

20 (a) Koilonychia.
(b) This is associated with iron-deficiency anaemia.

21 Mycosis fungoides. This is a disorder that presents initially as a non-specific scaly eruption, which eventually progresses with the formation of multiple skin tumours, some of which may ulcerate. The disease tends to affect middle-aged men and may be present for 20 years or more before it spreads systemically with lymphadenopathy and visceral involvement.

22 Xanthoma disseminatum.

23 Dermatomyositis. The illustration shows the classical heliotropic rash on the patient's face.

24 Synovial cyst.

25 Morphoea.

26 The *coup de sabre*. The diagnosis is once again morphoea.

27 Pressure necrosis of the skin.

28 Peutz–Jeghers syndrome.

29 (a) Dupuytren's contracture.
(b) This may be associated with other fibrotic conditions in the body, chronic alcoholism, and anticonvulsant therapy.

30 T1. The illustration shows small muscle wasting of the hands.

31 Pigmentation due to antimalarial agents. The pigmentatory disturbances include black pigmentation of the face, mucous membranes, and pretibial and subungual areas.

32 Chronic sarcoidosis (lupus pernio).

33 Prepatellar bursitis (housemaid's knee).

34 Polyarthritis due to lupus erythematosus. The photosensitive eruption on the dorsum of the hands is shown.

35 Primary osteoarthritis. This shows Heberden's nodes.

36 Still's disease.

37 Gouty tophi.

38 Dermatomyositis.

39 Sarcoidosis.

40 (a) High-arched palate associated with Marfan's syndrome.
(b) Ligament laxity should be sought, as well as evidence of lens dislocation, and mitral valve prolapse.

41 Scleroderma. There is evidence of sclerodactyly and terminal phalangeal gangrene.

42 She has beta thalassaemia major and has been receiving subcutaneous desferrioxamine, which caused the urine to turn yellow when the patient was eliminating iron.

43 Discoid lupus erythematosus. There is cicatricial alopecia and a scarred lesion on the face.

44 Pustulosis. No treatment was required, and the condition gradually subsided.

45 Ocular toxoplasmosis. An early choroidal lesion is shown.

46 The physical signs are those of dermatomyositis with nailfold vasculitic lesions and ragged cuticles.

47 Subungual fibroma due to tuberous sclerosis.

48 Chronic sarcoidosis. The picture shows some of the papular lesions characteristic of this condition.

49 Lingual thyroid.

50 (a) Keratoderma plantaris.
(b) This may be associated with Reiter's syndrome.

51 A thyroglossal cyst.

52 Strawberry naevus.

53 Pseudoxanthoma elasticum. Small yellowish papules forming linear or reticulate plaques, which in older people are soft, lax, and hang in folds, are distributed in the flexures, especially in the groins, axillae, and neck. The condition is associated with severe degeneration of Bruch's membrane, giving rise to the slate-grey, poorly defined angioid streaks, which form an incomplete ring of radiating lesions around the optic disc of the retina. The condition may also be associated with gastrointestinal bleeding.

54 Mongolian blue spots.

55 The generous hood of prepuce covers a severe hypospadias.

56 Urticaria pigmentosa. Mast cells are normally present in the skin, but the numbers vary greatly up to 80/mm³ in the upper dermis. In mastocytosis (urticaria pigmentosa) they are usually increased in number and may be found as a single isolated mastocytoma or numerous nests scattered over the entire body. Occasionally, there is systemic infiltration of all tissues including the liver, spleen, and bone marrow.

57 Keratosis pilaris.

58 Darier's disease. Nail signs may give a clue to the diagnosis, as demonstrated here. A white line extending from the nail bed to the distal nail plate, where there is a V-shaped notch, is characteristic. The disease is transmitted as a dominant gene.

59 Haemangioma.

60 Milroy's disease.

61 (a) Cutis laxa.
   (b) This is typical of Ehlers–Danlos syndrome.

62 (a) Syndactyly.
   (b) There are many syndromes associated with syndactyly, including congenital heart disease.

63 Ehlers–Danlos syndrome. This shows the cigarette-paper skin; classic of this condition.

64 Accessory toes.

65 Pectus excavatum.

66 This is a resection specimen of a polycystic kidney.

67 A gonad inside the labia.

68 Systemic mastocytosis.

69 Severe hypospadias.

70 Congenital adrenal hyperplasia with ambiguous genitalia.

71 Fordyce's spots.

72 Pectus carinatum (pigeon chest).

73 Diabetes mellitus. There has been an amputation of the little toe and there are some neuropathic ulcers.

74 Chondritis of the ear.

75 Spinocerebellar degeneration (Friedreich's ataxia). This disorder first begins in the legs in late childhood. The patient begins to stagger and lurch on walking and is unsteady on standing. Other features are clumsiness, a cerebellar tremor of the hands, dysarthria, and staccato speech. These symptoms result from changes in the dorsal root ganglia, the spinocerebellar tracts, and the cerebellum. The limbs also show considerable weakness, and skeletal deformities such as kyphoscoliosis occur. As in this picture, there is a peculiar foreshortening of the feet (pes cavus) with crooking of the toes, which is best ascribed to atrophy and contractures of the musculature of the feet at a time when the bones of the feet are malleable. Typically, there is a total absence of tendon reflexes and there are extensor plantar reflexes.

76 (a) Sabre tibia of Paget's disease.
(b) Raised serum alkaline phosphatase.

77 Graft versus host disease.

78 Gross surgical emphysema.

79 Hirsuties secondary to cyclosporin therapy.

80 Amiodarone-induced pigmentation.

81 Simple macular pigmentation.

82 Frostbite.

83 Argyria. Deposits of metal in the skin are seen, with silver where the skin appears blue–grey in colour. Gold (chrysiasis) where the skin has a brown to blue–grey colour, and clofazimine where the skin appears reddish-brown, are other caused of skin discoloration.

84 Lead poisoning. The discoloration of his gums is shown. Lead is a poison of enzymes, binding to the sulphydryl groups of proteins. It also interferes with calcium transport, the release of neurotransmitters, and activation of protein kinase. In high concentrations, lead alters the tertiary structure of intracellular proteins, denaturing them and causing cell death and tissue inflammation. The adult form of lead poisoning is characterized by abdominal pain, anaemia, renal disease, headache, peripheral neuropathy with demyelination of long neurons, ataxia, and memory loss.

85 (a) Erythema ab igne.
(b) This patient had been complaining of chronic abdominal pain and was using a hot water bottle to gain relief.

86 Dislocation of the lens.

87 Median nail dystrophy.

88 Impetigo.

89 Severe acanthosis nigricans. This is associated with severe insulin resistance.

90 (a) Alopecia areata.
(b) The patient should rub in some betamethasone ointment daily for a few weeks and the hair will generally regrow. An alternative solution would be to inject triamcinolone into the lesion.

91 Scleroderma. These are ischaemic ulcerated lesions.

92 Osler–Weber–Rendu disease (haemorrhagic telangiectasia).

93 (a) Acne comedones.
(b) This may be treated with an astringent cream or a keratolytic agent, such as benzoyl peroxide.

94 An aberrant left subclavian artery, causing dysphagia lusoria.

95 Central retinal artery occlusion.

96 This is a typical rash of glucagonoma, which is characteristically erythematous, raised, scaly, sometimes bullous and sometimes psoriatic, and ultimately crusted. It occurs primarily on the face, abdomen, perineum, and distal extremities. Patients with this condition may also have glossitis, stomatitis, angular cheilitis, dystrophic nails, and hair thinning. Weight loss, hypoaminoacidaemia, anaemia, and thromboembolic disease also occur.

97 Kaposi's sarcoma.

98 Conn's syndrome. The typical canary yellow coloration is shown.

99 Multiple fat emboli.

100 Kaposi's varicelliform eruption.

101 Generalized vasculitis, possibly due to polyarthritis nodosa.

102 Peutz–Jeghers syndrome. There is perioral pigmentation.

103 Sideroblastic anaemia. This shows ring sideroblasts.

104 Multiple laser coagulation scars in the eye of a diabetic.

105 (a) Target cells.
(b) These may occur post-splenectomy, in haemoglobinopathies, and in iron-deficiency anaemia.

106 There is severe osteopenia, but also anterior new bone formation. This is most characteristic of acromegaly.

107 Discoid lupus erythematosus.

108 Angioid streak. This may be seen in Paget's disease, sickle cell disease, and pseudoxanthoma elasticum.

109 Histiocytosis X.

110 (a) A keratopathy is shown and Bitot's spots are present.
(b) This is probably due to vitamin A deficiency.

111 Herpes genitalis.

112 Orf. These are the fingers of a farmer who works with sheep.

113 Toxic epidermal necrolysis.

114 Neurofibromatosis.

115 Central retinal artery occlusion. There is considerable oedema of the retina.

116 *Toxocara* infection of the eye.

117 Severe iron-deficiency anaemia. There is considerable aniso- and poikilocytosis. There are also occasional target cells and pencil cells.

118 Cold thyroid nodules. In this situation, there is a 10% chance of associated malignancy.

119 (a) Cytoid bodies.
(b) These may be associated with systemic lupus erythematosus.

120 Acute lymphoblastic leukaemia.

121 Crescenteric glomerulonephritis.

122 Thyroid acropachy. Clubbing of the fingers and toes with characteristic bone changes, which differ from those of hypertrophic pulmonary osteoarthropathy, may accompany the dermal changes (pretibial myxoedema) of thyroid acropachy.

123 Multiple myeloma.

124 Chronic myeloid leukaemia.

125 Exposure to asbestos. The chest radiograph shows some holly-leaf pleural plaques.

126 There is an infiltrate in both lungs with honeycombing. This is most typically seen in bronchiectasis, in this case due to cystic fibrosis. There is also a pneumothorax in the left hemithorax.

127 Atrial myxoma.

128 (a) Shortened fourth metacarpals, associated with pseudohypoparathyroidism.
(b) This is associated with a low serum calcium, a high phosphate, and a gross elevation of parathyroid hormone.

129 A Kimmelstiel–Wilson lesion is shown with a hyaline cap typical of diabetic nephropathy.

130 Urticarial vasculitis. This may occasionally be associated with thyrotoxicosis.

131 The most likely diagnosis is metabolic bone disease, in this case due to vitamin D deficiency. There is a generalized increase in uptake, with multiple hot spots due to small fractures.

132 Sclerolimbic calcification, typical of hypercalcaemia.

133 (a) There is a gross pituitary mass.
(b) The visual fields should be inspected for evidence of a bitemporal field defect.

134 (a) Central section magnetic resonance imaging (MRI) scan.
(b) There is an enlarged pituitary, which is barely touching the optic chiasm.

135 Pointing empyema necessitans. The patient had a tuberculous empyema.

136 Hashimoto's thyroiditis. This shows granulomas and lymphocytic aggregates, as well as scarring and destruction of the thyroid parenchyma.

137 There is a thyroid mass with tracheal deviation on this computerized tomography (CT) scan of the neck.

138 The ovary is slightly enlarged, and clearly shows multiple subcapsular cysts. This appearance is typical of the polycystic ovary syndrome.

139 This is a typical neuropathic ulcer in a diabetic.

140 This is a muscle biopsy showing a normal distribution of type I and type II muscle fibres.

141 Posterior subcapsular cataract.

142 Pyoderma gangrenosum.

143 Acrodermatitis enteropathica. In this disease zinc deficiency may be due to a defect in zinc absorption. The onset of symptoms often occurs when an affected infant is weaned from human milk to cow's milk. In zinc deficiency, tissues with a high cellular turnover, including skin, gastrointestinal mucosa, chondrocytes, spermatogonia, and thymocytes are characteristically affected. The dermatological manifestations (hyperkeratosis, parakeratosis, acrodermatitis, and alopecia) evoke the possibility of zinc deficiency. The usual distribution of the keratotic lesions is in areas that are readily traumatized, such as the elbows and knees. The keratotic lesions can become pustular or develop into crusting, red, scaly plaques.

144 Stevens–Johnson syndrome.

145 Behçet's disease.

146 Pemphigoid.

147 Burns' contractures.

148 Penicillamine-induced pemphigus.

149 (a) Shortened fourth metacarpal.
(b) This may be found in Kallmann's syndrome as well as in pseudo-hypoparathyroidism.

150 Paraganglionomas, with a skull vault metastasis. This is a metaiodo-benzylguanidine (MIBG) scan. MIBG is a chromaffin-seeking compound from a derivative of guanethidine, which will often help localize abnormal chromaffin tissue, as in this case.

151 Ruptured rectus sheath with haematoma.

152 Coeliac disease. The classic subtotal villous atrophy is clearly shown.

153 Capital alopecia of secondary syphilis.

154 (a) This is a transabdominal ultrasound.
(b) It shows the bladder and a polycystic ovary with a bright parenchymal echo and subcapsular 5–7 mm cysts.

155 Galactorrhoea is shown. This may be caused by a prolactinoma or the use of a dopamine antagonist, such as a phenothiazine.

156 Advanced diabetic retinopathy with scar formation due to retinitis proliferans.

157 (a) Bilateral gynaecomastia.
(b) This is probably related to his obesity, but if glandular tissue is palpable, oestrogen levels should be measured and thyroid function tested. His testes should be examined carefully for the possibility of a Leydig cell tumour.

158 *Candida* infection of the skin. This shows crusted satellite lesions.

159 A dopamine agonist has been given to shrink a prolactin-secreting macroadenoma of the pituitary.

160 Adenoma sebaceum (Bourneville–Becker disease).

161 Gross pretibial myxoedema (hypertrophic/hyperkeratotic variant).

162 Scleroderma. The nose is pinched, and telangiectatic lesions are visible. Puckering of the upper lip is also evident.

163 This is a methylene bisphosphonate bone scan showing up hot spots in a patient with Paget's disease.

164 Pretibial myxoedema.

165 He is grossly hypogonadal and probably has Kallmann's syndrome together with X-linked ichthyosis, a contiguous gene defect knocking out two genes on the $Xp_{22.3}$ part of the genome.

166 Multiple strictures, probably due to Crohn's disease.

167 Dysphagia. This is the imprint left by an anomalous subclavian artery.

168 Pretibial myxoedema.

169 Cushing's syndrome. Her facial plethora and hirsuties are shown.

170 Bazin's erythema induratum (tuberculosis).

171 Squamous carcinoma of the skin.

172 Fixed drug eruption.

173 Livedo reticularis. This may be seen with polyarteritis nodosa.

174 Acute glaucoma. Oedema of the cornea is seen.

175 Lupus vulgaris.

176 Necrobiosis lipoidica diabeticorum.

177 Disciform macular degeneration.

178 Carcinoid syndrome. In the long term, these patients can develop tryptophan deficiency and develop pellagra.

179 (a) Arachnodactyly.
(b) This may be associated with Marfan's syndrome and Ehlers–Danlos syndrome.

180 Dermatomyositis.

181 Scrofula. This is the appearance of multiple, previously discharging tuberculous lymph nodes.

182 Lupus pernio (sarcoidosis).

183 Polycystic ovary syndrome. There is hirsuties and mild acne. Other features include capital hair loss, greasy skin, oligomenorrhoea, and the typical polycystic appearances of the ovaries.

184 There is an irregular pupil, an iridectomy operation has been performed, and there is a subconjunctival haemorrhage.

185 Congenital cyanotic heart disease.

186 This is retinitis pigmentosa, which may have been caused in this case by chronic phenothiazine intake.

187 Retinal detachment.

188 Basal cell carcinoma.

189 Melanoma with metastatic lesions.

190 Metastatic lesion of the liver. The left adrenal gland is also abnormal.

191 Pseudoxanthoma elasticum.

192 These are counter-irritation (cigarette burn) marks, and are a traditional tribal therapy for chronic abdominal pain.

193 (a) Bilateral gynaecomastia.
(b) This may occasionally occur physiologically during puberty. However, in this situation, it is marked, and the patient should be examined for actual glandular tissue of the breast. His testes should also be examined carefully. The drugs that can cause gynaecomastia include digoxin, cimetidine, spironolactone, and cyproterone acetate.

194 Still's disease.

195 (a) This is a radioisotope renogram.
(b) It shows delayed passage of radionucleotide in one of the kidneys. This is typical of renovascular disease.

196 XYY karyotype (not Klinefelter's XXY).

197 Heterochromia iridis.

198 Gross myxoedema.

199 Erythema nodosum.

200 Chilblains (perniosis).

INDEX

Numbers refer to Question and Answer numbers.

empyema necessitans, 135
erythema:
  Bazin's erythema induratum, 170
  erythema ab igne, 85
  erythema nodosum, 199
eye:
  cataract, 141
  glaucoma, 174
  heterochromia iridis, 197
  irregular pupil, 184
  keratopathy, 110
  laser coagulation scars, 104
  lens dislocation, 86
  macular degeneration, 177
  macular pigmentation, 81
  multiple fat emboli, 99
  ocular toxoplasmosis, 45
  sclerolimbic calcification, 132
  subconjunctival haemorrhage, 184
  Toxocara infection, 116
  see also retina

facial plethora, 169
feet:
  accessory toes, 64
  Charcot's joints, 12
  frostbite, 82
  keratoderma plantaris, 50
  neuropathic ulcers, 73
  spinocerebellar degeneration, 75
fibroma, subungual, 47
fingers *see* hands
fixed drug eruption, 172
Fordyce's spots, 71
Friedreich's ataxia, 75
frostbite, 82

galactorrhoea, 155
gangrene, terminal phalangeal, 41
genitalia, ambiguous, 67, 70
glandular fever, 19
glaucoma, 174
glomerulonephritis, 121
glucagonoma, 96
gonococcal infection, 2
gouty tophi, 37
graft versus host disease, 77
granulomas, 136
gynaecomastia, 157, 193

haemangioma, 59
haematoma, 151
haemorrhagic telangiectasia, 92

hand, foot, and mouth disease, 17
hands:
  arachnodactyly, 179
  chilblains, 200
  dermatomyositis, 38, 46
  Dupuytren's contracture, 29
  gonococcal infection, 2
  hyperkeratosis palmaris, 5
  metacarpal shortening, 128, 149
  osteoarthritis, 35
  polyarthritis, 34
  sarcoidosis, 16
  scleroderma, 41, 91
  small muscle wasting, 30
  Still's disease, 194
  synovial cyst, 24
  toxic epidermal necrolysis, 113
  see also nails
Hashimoto's thyroiditis, 136
Heberden's nodes, 35
Herpes genitalis, 111
heterochromia iridis, 197
high-arched palate, 40
hirsuties, 79, 169, 183
histiocytosis X, 109
holly-leaf pleural plaques, 125
housemaid's knee, 33
Hutchinson's teeth, 14
hypercalcaemia, 11, 132
hyperkeratosis palmaris, 5
hypospadias, 55, 69

impetigo, 88
insulin resistance, 89
iridectomy, 184
iron deficiency anaemia, 20, 102, 117

joints, Charcot's, 12

Kallmann's syndrome, 149, 165
Kaposi's sarcoma, 97
Kaposi's varicelliform eruption, 100
keratoderma plantaris, 50
keratopathy, 110
keratosis pilaris, 57
kidney, polycystic, 66
Kimmelstiel–Wilson lesion, 129
koilonychia, 20

lead poisoning, 84
leukaemia:
  mphoblastic, 120
  myeloid, 124